Lisa Monroe, .

Preventing Glaucoma

How to Take Care of Your Eyes

First edition

This book was professionally typeset on Reedsy
Find out more at reedsy.com

This book is dedicated to all those looking to effectively manage glaucoma.

Contents

1.

2.

3.

4.

5.

6.

7.

8.

9.

10.

11.

12.

13.

14.

15.

16.

17.

18.

19.

20.

21.

Acknowledgement

Special thanks to God, the Publisher, and the Editor for their immense contributions and support in completing this masterpiece.

I

Introduction

1

Understanding Glaucoma

Understanding Glaucoma

Glaucoma is described as an expanded strain inside the eye, which can harm the optic nerve and cause long-lasting vision misfortune. Glaucoma is frequently alluded to as the "quiet criminal of sight," since it commonly has no side effects in its beginning phases and can go undetected for quite a long time.

The reasons for glaucoma are not completely understood, yet it is accepted that the condition is brought about by a blend of hereditary and ecological elements. Some risk factors for glaucoma include age, family ancestry, high eye pressure, and certain ailments like diabetes.

There are a few sorts of glaucoma, including open-point glaucoma, point conclusion glaucoma, and typical pressure glaucoma. Open-point glaucoma is the most widely recognized type, representing around 90% of all cases. This kind of glaucoma grows slowly and ordinarily has no side effects until it has proactively caused huge vision misfortune. Conclusion: Glaucoma, then again, grows rapidly and can cause serious eye agony, migraines, and vision misfortune. Ordinary strain glaucoma happens when there is optic nerve damage and vision misfortune, despite the fact that eye pressure is within the typical range.

The objective of glaucoma treatment is to forestall further harm to the optic nerve and protect vision. Treatment choices change contingent upon the kind and seriousness of glaucoma; however, they may incorporate eye drops, oral medications, laser medical procedures, or conventional medical procedures.

Eye drops are normally the principal line of treatment for open-point glaucoma. These drops work by decreasing eye pressure and working on the progression of liquid out of the eye. It is critical to use eye drops as endorsed by a specialist, as missing portions or halting treatment rashly can bring about additional vision misfortune.

At times, oral prescriptions might be endorsed notwithstanding or rather than eye drops. These medications work by lessening eye pressure and working on the progression of liquid out of the eye. It is vital to educate a specialist regarding some other medications being taken, as certain drugs can interact with glaucoma medications.

Laser medical procedures are in many cases used to treat both open-ended and closed-point glaucoma. In this system, a laser is utilized to make minuscule openings in the trabecular meshwork, the region of the eye that directs liquid outpouring. This assists with diminishing eye pressure and forestalls further optic nerve harm.

Conventional medical procedures might be vital for serious instances of glaucoma that don't respond to different therapies. In this technique, a specialist makes another channel for liquid to drain out of the eye, bypassing the hindered or damaged regions.

Notwithstanding these medicines, lifestyle changes can likewise assist with overseeing glaucoma. These may include keeping a sound eating regimen, practicing routinely, and staying away from exercises that increase eye pressure, like lifting weighty items or stressing to go to the washroom.

Customary eye tests are fundamental for recognizing and treating glaucoma early.

2

Causes

Glaucoma is a group of eye conditions that can cause irreversible visual impairment if left untreated. It is described by high tension inside the eye, which harms the optic nerve and, bit by bit, lessens vision. While there is no single reason for glaucoma, there are a few factors that can contribute to its development. Let's talk about the most widely recognized reasons for glaucoma and their effect on eye wellbeing.

1. Age

As individuals become older, the risk of developing glaucoma increases. This is on the grounds that the normal waste framework inside the eye turns out to be less productive with age, prompting an expansion in intraocular pressure. Thus, people beyond 40 years old must have normal eye tests to distinguish any indications of glaucoma from the get-go.

2. Hereditary qualities

Glaucoma can likewise be brought about by hereditary qualities. People who have a family history of the illness are at a higher risk of creating it themselves. Now and again, glaucoma can be acquired as an autosomal dominant attribute, implying that the quality responsible for the condition can be passed down starting with one age and then onto the next. Hereditary testing can assist with distinguishing people who are in danger of developing glaucoma and recommending early mediation.

3. Eye wounds

Eye wounds, like a disaster for the eye or an infiltrating injury, can prompt glaucoma. This is on the grounds that these wounds can disturb the normal waste framework inside the eye and cause strain. It is critical to seek clinical consideration right away, assuming that you experience any kind of eye injury, to forestall any expected long-term harm to your vision.

4. Meds

Certain medications, like corticosteroids, can cause an expansion of intraocular strain and lead to glaucoma. This is particularly true for people who are taking these drugs for a long time or in large portions. Assuming that you are taking any prescription and notice any progressions in your vision or experience any distress in your eyes, talk with your medical services supplier to decide whether the medicine could be the reason.

5. Medical Conditions

A few ailments can increase the chance of creating glaucoma. These circumstances incorporate diabetes, hypertension, and hypothyroidism. Assuming you have any of these circumstances, it is essential to inform your eye specialist with the goal that they can screen your eye wellbeing all the more intently.

6. Ethnicity

Certain ethnic groups are more vulnerable to developing glaucoma than others. For instance, African Americans and people of Hispanic descent are at a higher risk of developing open-point glaucoma, the most widely recognized type of the condition. This is on the grounds that they will generally have a more slender cornea, which can prompt a mistaken intraocular pressure reading and a deferred conclusion.

While there is no explicit cause for glaucoma, a few variables can add to its turn of events.

3

Symptoms

The symptoms of glaucoma can shift depending on the kind of glaucoma and the phase of the infection. Notwithstanding, there are a few normal side effects that are often present in people with this condition. One of the most outstanding side effects is vision misfortune. This can happen in one or both eyes and can be continuous or abrupt. Many individuals with glaucoma additionally experience limited focus, where their fringe vision is seriously confined, making it hard to see objects.

Other side effects of glaucoma include eye agony, redness, and obscured vision. Certain individuals may likewise notice that their eyes seem shady or dim. These side effects are many times more recognizable during times of expanded tension in the eye, for example, during demanding movement or after an extensive stretch of sitting.

At times, people with glaucoma may likewise encounter side effects connected with their actual wellbeing. For instance, they might have cerebral pain, feel sick, or experience tipsiness. These side effects can be connected with changes in the blood stream or changes in the body's hormonal equilibrium, both of which can be impacted by glaucoma.

There are a few distinct kinds of glaucoma, each with its own unique side effects and causes. The most well-known structure is open-point glaucoma, which happens when the waste channels in the eye become obstructed, causing tension in the eye. This kind of glaucoma is regularly effortless and causes no observable side effects until critical harm has been done to the optic nerve.

Point conclusion Glaucoma, then again, is more extreme and can cause unexpected side effects, including serious eye torment, sickness, heaving, and an unexpected diminishing in vision. This kind of glaucoma happens when the iris obstructs the waste trenches in the eye, making pressure build up quickly. This is a health-related crisis and requires prompt treatment to forestall this extremely durable vision misfortune.

There are a few risk factors for glaucoma, including age, family ancestry, and certain ailments like diabetes. African Americans and Hispanics are likewise at a higher risk of developing glaucoma than other ethnic groups.

Treatment choices for glaucoma are contingent upon the sort and seriousness of the sickness. The objective of treatment is to lessen tension in the eye and forestall further harm to the optic nerve. This can be accomplished through medicine, laser treatment, or a medical procedure. Prescriptions, for example, eye drops, are normally the principal line of treatment for glaucoma, as they can actually decrease strain in the eye without bringing on any huge secondary effects.

Laser therapy is another choice and includes utilizing a powerful light emission to decrease tension in the eye.

4

Risk Factors

Glaucoma is an ever-evolving eye condition that harms the optic nerve and prompts irreversible visual deficiency on the off chance that it is not recognized and treated early. It is the subsequent driving reason for visual deficiency universally and influences a great many individuals around the world. A few variables increase the risk of creating glaucoma, including age, hereditary qualities, ailments, and way of life decisions.

Age is a huge risk factor for glaucoma, and it normally influences individuals north of 40 years of age. The risk of fostering the condition increases as one ages, and individuals north of 60 years of age are multiple times more likely to foster glaucoma than those in their 40s. Age-related eye changes, like a reduction in fluid humor surge and the development of strain, contribute to the improvement of glaucoma. Individuals north of 40 years of age ought to get an exhaustive eye test routinely to screen their eye wellbeing and distinguish early indications of glaucoma.

Hereditary qualities play a fundamental role in the improvement of glaucoma. In the event that one has a family history of glaucoma, the risk of fostering the condition is higher. A few qualities are related to various kinds of glaucoma, like essential open-point glaucoma and essential innate glaucoma. Individuals with a family history of glaucoma ought to consult their eye specialist to seek early screening and treatment.

Certain ailments additionally increase the risk of creating glaucoma. Individuals with diabetes are bound to develop glaucoma because of changes in veins that influence eye capability. Other ailments that can increase the risk of glaucoma include hypertension, coronary illness, and headaches. Individuals with these circumstances ought to get normal eye tests to distinguish early indications of glaucoma.

Lifestyle decisions like smoking, high liquor utilization, and a terrible eating routine can likewise increase the risk of glaucoma. Smoking increases intraocular strain and harms the optic nerve, prompting glaucoma. Liquor utilization can increase eye pressure and diminish blood flow to the optic nerve, prompting glaucoma. An eating routine high in saturated fats and processed food varieties can likewise increase the risk of glaucoma. Individuals ought to abstain from smoking, limit liquor utilization, and maintain a solid eating regimen to decrease their risk of glaucoma.

Other risk factors for glaucoma include eye wounds, constant steroid use, and ethnicity. Eye wounds that harm the optic nerve or increase eye strain can prompt glaucoma. Long-term utilization of steroids can increase intraocular tension and cause glaucoma. Certain ethnic groups, like African Americans and Hispanics, are bound to foster glaucoma more than Caucasians. These groups ought to get ordinary eye tests to identify early indications of glaucoma.

Glaucoma is a dynamic eye condition that influences a huge number of individuals around the world. A few risk factors improve the probability of developing glaucoma, including age, hereditary qualities, ailments, and way of life decisions. Individuals ought to get ordinary eye tests to screen their eye health and identify early indications of glaucoma.

5

Importance of early detection and prevention

While the actual infection can't be relieved, it tends to be managed successfully with early discovery and treatment. Subsequently, it is of principal significance to recognize glaucoma as soon as possible to forestall the advancement of the infection and to keep up with the wellbeing of the eyes.

One of the essential explanations behind the significance of early identification of glaucoma is the fact that the illness is generally asymptomatic in its beginning phases. Numerous patients might have glaucoma without encountering any perceptible side effects. As such, you might have glaucoma and not even know it! In the event that the sickness slips by everyone's notice for a really long time, nonetheless, it can prompt extremely durable vision misfortune. Normal eye tests with your optometrist or ophthalmologist are urgent to catch the infection almost immediately and keep it from bringing about additional harm.

Notwithstanding the asymptomatic idea of early glaucoma, it is vital to consider the risk factors for fostering the illness. These risk factors incorporate age, family ancestry, nationality, and ailments like diabetes and hypertension. While you have zero control over your age or family ancestry, you can deal with the other risk factors by embracing a solid way of life and visiting your eye specialist routinely. With early identification, you can work with your medical services supplier to deal with your risk factors and forestall the advancement of glaucoma.

Early recognition of glaucoma likewise empowers early treatment, which is fundamental for keeping solid eyes. There are different treatment options accessible for glaucoma, contingent upon the seriousness of the infection and the patient's extraordinary conditions. Meds, laser treatment, and medical procedures are normal therapies for glaucoma. By identifying the illness early, patients have a superior chance of protecting their vision with the least intrusive treatment conceivable.

The prevention of glaucoma is likewise conceivable through early identification. While there is no dependable method for keeping glaucoma from growing, early recognition can assist patients in recognizing and dealing with the risk factors for the sickness. Overseeing circulatory strain and glucose levels, keeping a sound eating regimen and workout schedule, and safeguarding the eyes from UV beams are all instances of steps that patients can take to reduce their risk of developing glaucoma. Early discovery and the use of these gamble variables can diminish the probability of creating glaucoma later on.

Early discovery and counteraction of glaucoma can fundamentally affect a patient's personal satisfaction. Vision misfortune can significantly affect a person's freedom, capacity to work, and general personal satisfaction. Early discovery and treatment can forestall these adverse consequences and assist patients with maintaining their autonomy and personal satisfaction into the indefinite future.

Early identification and counteraction of glaucoma are of the utmost significance for keeping up with the soundness of the eyes and forestalling vision misfortune.

II

Healthy Habits

6

Tips for maintaining good eye health

As we go through our day-to-day schedules, we will generally disregard the significance of our vision. It is a gift that we frequently underestimate, not understanding how fundamental it is for us to play out our errands, complete our everyday exercises, and explore our strategy for getting around. Thus, it is significant to keep up with great eye wellbeing to stay away from any unfavorable effect on our eyes. Here are a few hints to keep your eyes in great shape and your vision really sharp.

Eat Healthily:

The food that you eat is quite possibly one of the most basic variables that influence your general wellbeing. For better eye wellbeing, consolidate a solid eating regimen into your daily schedule. Eating an eating routine that is rich in green, verdant vegetables like spinach and kale and different vegetables like carrots, yams, pumpkin, and so on. will guarantee that your eyes are all around fed. Fish, which are wealthy in omega-3 unsaturated fats like salmon, fish, and halibut, can likewise be exceptionally valuable.

Limit Screen Time:

The period of mechanical progression has brought about expanded screen time and, in this manner, an ascent in computerized eye strain, migraines, and eye weariness. Whether it's for work, mingling, or diversion purposes, attempt to restrict your screen time and observe the 20-20-20 guideline, which is to screen at regular intervals, take a 20-second break, and turn away 20 feet. This standard permits your eyes to unwind, decreasing the probability of eye exhaustion and inconvenience.

Use Eye Protection:

Involving eye assurance in different situations can assist with keeping up with great eye wellbeing. When out in the sun, it is crucial to wear shades to shield your eyes from destructive UV beams, which can harm your retina and cause waterfalls. Essentially, while working with unsafe materials, defensive eyewear like goggles, safeguards, and wellbeing glasses ought to be worn to forestall eye injury.

Get Sufficient Rest:

Getting satisfactory rest is significant for your general wellbeing, and it is the same with regards to keeping up with great eye wellbeing. Absence of rest can cause eye exhaustion, strain, and other related issues like dry eyes. Ensure you get no less than seven to eight hours of rest to rest your eyes and keep up with ideal eye wellbeing.

Stay Hydrated:

Lack of hydration can cause eye strain, obscured vision, and dry eyes. It is vital to drink a lot of water to maintain ideal eye health. Drinking a satisfactory measure of water assists with keeping up with the creation of tears, which keep your eyes damp.

Work-out Routinely:

Exercise can advance the course all through the body, including the eyes. Normal activity can assist with preventing different eye issues, for example, glaucoma and age-related macular degeneration, among others. Activities, for example, yoga and reflection, can likewise assist with loosening up the eyes and lessening eye weakness and strain.

Regular Eye Check-ups:

Getting standard eye tests is crucial for maintaining good eye health.

7

Nutrition for eye health

Nutrition is fundamental for maintaining solid vision and preventing eye issues. There are different kinds of food varieties and supplements that play a fundamental role in advancing eye wellbeing. Appropriate nourishment can shield the eyes from a few issues, for example, waterfalls, age-related macular degeneration, and other vision hindrances. Let's look at some of the best foods and supplements that can uphold and work on your vision.

Carrots are the main food that strikes a chord with regards to eye wellbeing. This is on the grounds that carrots contain beta-carotene, a forerunner of vitamin A. Vitamin A is a fundamental supplement that keeps up with legitimate eye capabilities. It helps in framing the retinal color and keeping the outer layer of the eye clammy. Devouring carrots and other food sources abundant in vitamin A can forestall dry eyes and shield the eyes from different eye contaminations.

Spinach is another supplement-rich food that can altogether improve sound and visual perception. It contains two fundamental supplements, lutein and zeaxanthin. These supplements have been shown to lessen the risk of age-related macular degeneration. The macula is the piece of the retina that gives sharp, focal vision. By eating food varieties like spinach that are high in these two supplements, you can safeguard the macula and forestall vision misfortune.

Blueberries are known for their cell-reinforcement properties and their various medical advantages. They are likewise perfect for eye health. Blueberries are rich in anthocyanins, which help in further developing vision and decreasing the risk of cataracts and glaucoma. These strong cancer prevention agents shield the eye from oxidative pressure and decrease aggravation in the retina.

Nuts and seeds, for example, almonds, sunflower seeds, and peanuts, are incredible wellsprings of vitamin E, a strong cell reinforcement that safeguards the eyes from oxidative pressure. This kind of pressure is brought about by free extremists, which are temperamental atoms that can harm the cells in the eyes. By devouring food sources abundant in vitamin E, you can forestall the improvement of cataracts and age-related macular degeneration.

Fish like salmon, tuna, and mackerel are high in omega-3 unsaturated fats. Omega-3s are fundamental unsaturated fats that are expected to keep up with sound vision. They assist in preventing dry eyes, which can cause eye irritation and different confusions. Omega-3s are likewise helpful in lessening irritation in the eyes, which is a main source of many eye illnesses.

Green tea is an extraordinary refreshment to add to your eating routine if you have any desire to work on your vision. Green tea contains strong cell reinforcements known as catechins, which are accepted to forestall age-related macular degeneration. Drinking green tea routinely can assist with shielding the eyes from UV beams and diminishing irritation.

It's additionally vital to limit your utilization of handled food sources, sweet tidbits, and other food sources high in undesirable fats. These food varieties can increase your risk of developing eye issues and other unexpected problems.

8

Exercises to strengthen eyes

As we invest increasingly more energy gazing at screens and other electronic gadgets, it's no big surprise that eye strain and vision issues are on the rise. Yet, fortunately, there are basic activities you can do to assist with reinforcing your eyes and keeping them good for quite a long time into the future. Here are probably the best activities to fortify your eyes:

1. Eye rolling

This exercise is basically as straightforward as it sounds. Basically, feign exacerbation in a round movement, first in one course and afterward in the other. This assists with reinforcing the muscles around your eyes and can ease pressure and weariness.

2. Eye focus

Hold your thumb out at a careful distance and shine a spotlight on it. Gradually carry your thumb nearer to your face, actually zeroing in on it, until it is around three creeps from your nose. Then, at that point, gradually move it back on a mission to a safe distance. Rehash this exercise a couple of times, enjoying reprieves on the off chance that your eyes feel stressed.

3. Near and far focus

Pick a far-off object to zero in on, then center around a nearer object. Do this to and fro for a couple of moments, again enjoying reprieves if necessary. This assists with practicing the muscles responsible for changing the focal point of your eyes.

4. Blinking

It might appear like an easy decision, but flickering is really a significant activity for your eyes. It assists with keeping your eyes greased up and prevents dryness and irritation. Attempt to flicker all the more regularly, particularly while gazing at evaluations for expanded timeframes.

5. Palming

This assists with loosening up your eyes and lessening strain and pressure.

6. Figure-eight eye development

Picture a nonexistent figure eight about ten feet from you. Then, at that point, follow the figure eight with your eyes, moving your look without a hitch and consistently from one side to the next. This exercise can assist with further developing eye coordination and muscle strength.

7. Up and down eye movement

Turn upward to the furthest extent that you would be able, then peer down to the furthest extent that you would be able. Rehash this exercise a couple of times, enjoying reprieves on the off chance that your eyes feel stressed. This assists with practicing the muscles responsible for vertical eye development.

8. Letter tracking

Pick a letter on a page, then, at that point, follow it with your eyes as smoothly and consistently as you can. Rehash this activity with various letters, numbers, or images on the page. This assists with further developing eye coordination and muscle strength.

9. Focus on details

Pick a little item with fine subtleties, similar to a coin or a button, and shine a spotlight on it for a couple of moments. Attempt to consider every one of the subtleties as plainly as could be expected. This exercise can assist with working on your capacity to see fine subtleties.

10. PC breaks

On the off chance that you invest a ton of energy gazing at a PC screen, enjoy continuous reprieves to give your eyes a rest.

9

Importance of regular eye check-ups

As people, our visual perception is quite possibly our most valuable gift. It is our primary wellspring of tangible data, permitting us to encounter our general surroundings in the entirety of their magnificence and multifaceted nature. Nonetheless, many individuals underestimate their vision and don't focus on customary eye check-ups, prompting undetected vision issues that can have enduring and adverse impacts. Standard eye check-ups are vital in light of the fact that they assist with recognizing vision issues that we could not in any case notice. Frequently, vision changes happen bit by bit and slip through the cracks until they arrive at a high-level stage, making them more difficult to address. For example, vision changes related to conditions, such as glaucoma and waterfalls, might be irreversible, bringing about long-lasting vision misfortune. Nonetheless, early location and treatment can forestall or defer the beginning of such vision issues, making it more straightforward to oversee and possibly even reverse certain circumstances. Moreover, ordinary eye check-ups can likewise assist with distinguishing fundamental medical issues, for example, diabetes and hypertension, which can adversely affect our vision.

Besides, standard eye check-ups are fundamental for keeping up with general eye wellbeing. During a far-reaching eye test, an optometrist or ophthalmologist checks for normal eye illnesses and conditions, including dry eye disorder, conjunctivitis, and macular degeneration, among others. By checking changes in your vision and looking at the strength of your eyes, a certified eye specialist can assist you with distinguishing any irregularities that require clinical consideration, give direction on treatment choices, and prompt you on advances you can take to forestall further decay. They can likewise suggest defensive measures, for example, wearing shades or eye safeguards to protect your eyes from the sun or trash, which can harm the cornea or the retina.

Another justification for why normal eye check-ups are significant is that they can save you cash and time over the long haul. It is significantly more financially savvy and time-effective to forestall and distinguish issues from the get-go as opposed to overseeing more serious vision issues that require escalated medicines. Customary check-ups may appear to be a burden, yet the expected expenses and lost time due to dismissing your visual wellbeing are considerably more significant. Actually, without appropriate eye care, you risk harming your visual perception forever and, conceivably, in any event, requiring an exorbitant eye medical procedure.

Past forestalling or overseeing eye issues, normal eye check-ups offer various advantages, for example, assisting you with benefiting from your restorative eyewear, working on visual execution, and helping in general eye wellbeing. Assuming you wear eyeglasses or contact lenses, standard check-ups can assist you with keeping up with their adequacy. It is clear and agreeable to guarantee your vision. Additionally, some vision issues, like presbyopia, can be resolved with contact focal points and moderate focal points. Accordingly, you ought to counsel your optometrist to find out about accessible focal point choices and find out which would best accommodate your way of life.

Regular eye check-ups offer an inward feeling of harmony and work on personal satisfaction.

III

Glaucoma Prevention Strategies

10

Medication management for those at risk

As the familiar proverb goes, avoidance is superior to fixing. This is particularly valid for those in danger of developing glaucoma, an ever-evolving illness that harms the optic nerve and can prompt vision misfortune or visual deficiency whenever left untreated. Luckily, medicine can assist with decreasing the risk of creating glaucoma or slowing its movement.

There are various kinds of glaucoma; however, the most well-known one is open-point glaucoma, which is in many cases brought about by raised intraocular pressure (IOP). The primary line of defense against glaucoma is to diminish IOP, which can be accomplished through drugs that increase seepage or decrease the creation of watery humor, the liquid in the eye.

Below are the primary classes of glaucoma medications:

Prostaglandin analogs: these drugs are viewed as the best option for glaucoma treatment because of their adequacy and accommodation. They work by expanding the outpouring of watery humor through the trabecular meshwork, which diminishes IOP. Models incorporate latanoprost (Xalatan), bimatoprost (Lumigan), and travoprost (Travatan Z).

Beta blockers: these drugs diminish the development of watery humor by obstructing the activity of beta-adrenergic receptors. They are likewise compelling at bringing down IOP, but they are contraindicated in patients with specific ailments like asthma and coronary illness. Models incorporate timolol (Timoptic), betaxolol (Betoptic), and levobunolol (Betagan).

Alpha agonists: these medications lessen the creation of watery humor and increase its outpouring by choking the veins in the eye. They are typically utilized as second-line specialists because of their side effects like dry mouth and weakness. Models incorporate brimonidine (Alphagan P) and apraclonidine (Iopidine).

Carbonic anhydrase inhibitors: these medications lessen the development of watery humor by hindering the activity of carbonic anhydrase, a compound engaged with the arrangement of the liquid. They are accessible as eye drops or oral tablets; however, the last option can cause more foundational side effects. Models incorporate dorzolamide (Trusopt) and brinzolamide (Azopt).

Rho kinase inhibitors: these medications are a more current class of glaucoma sedates that increment the surge of fluid humor by loosening up the trabecular meshwork. They are regularly utilized as extra treatment for patients who have not achieved an adequate IOP decrease with different medications. The main endorsed prescription in this class is netarsudil (Rhopressa).

Combination meds: these are eye drops that contain at least two classes of glaucoma drugs, which can help with drug organization and lessen the risk of secondary effects from various prescriptions. Models incorporate dorzolamide-timolol (Cosopt) and brimonidine-timolol (Combigan).

11

Surgery and other medical treatments

Fortunately, there are different treatment options accessible to patients experiencing this condition.

One of the most well-known medicines for glaucoma is the utilization of prescriptions, for example, eye drops, which work to bring down the intraocular pressure. These prescriptions can be utilized in various mixes and might be recommended for long-term use. They are successful in dealing with the condition and forestalling its movement.

Nonetheless, now and again, medicine alone may not be adequate for controlling intraocular pressure. In such cases, careful mediation might be vital. The two most common and safe medicines for glaucoma are trabeculectomy and tube shunting, a medical procedure.

Trabeculectomy is a surgery that includes making a little fold in the sclera (the white piece of the eye), which permits liquid to stream out of the eye and lower the intraocular pressure. This technique is finished under neighborhood sedation and may require a couple of long stretches of hospitalization for post-use consideration. The achievement pace of this system is high, with most patients attaining typical intraocular pressure levels. Be that as it may, there might be a few incidental effects, like waterfall development, and patients might have to keep utilizing medicine to control the condition.

A tube shunt is a medical procedure that, again, includes setting a little cylinder in the eye, which permits liquid to stream out of the eye and lower the intraocular pressure. This cylinder is associated with a repository, which is embedded behind the eye. This methodology is likewise completed under neighborhood sedation and may require a couple of long stretches of hospitalization for post-usable consideration. The achievement pace of this strategy is likewise high, with most patients attaining ordinary intraocular pressure levels. In any case, as with trabeculectomy, there might be a few secondary effects, like waterfall development.

Both of these methodologies are exceptionally compelling in treating glaucoma; however, they may not be appropriate for everybody. Your eye specialist will evaluate your condition and decide on the most fitting treatment for you.

Notwithstanding medical procedures, there are different therapies accessible for glaucoma, like laser medical procedures and negligibly intrusive glaucoma medical procedures (MIGS). Laser medical procedures include utilizing an extraordinary kind of laser to bring down the intraocular strain by opening up the waste diverts in the eye. This technique is based on a short-term premise and is surprisingly easy. MIGS, then again, is a somewhat new sort of glaucoma medical procedure that utilizes minuscule gadgets to decrease intraocular pressure. These gadgets are embedded in the eye and attempt to work on liquid surge.

There are different treatment choices accessible for patients experiencing glaucoma, ranging from drugs to careful intervention.

12

Laser surgery for Glaucoma

The conventional treatment strategies incorporate prescription and careful mediation, yet one present-day treatment choice acquiring ubiquity is the laser medical procedure.

Laser medical procedures are a painless system that is speedy, protected, and powerful in treating glaucoma. The methodology works by utilizing a high-energy laser to lessen how much liquid is created in the eye, which thus brings down the eye pressure that is brought about by the overabundance of liquid development. By bringing down the eye pressure, laser medical procedures can diminish the harm caused to the optic nerve by glaucoma and forestall further loss of vision.

The advantages of laser medical procedures for glaucoma are huge. The system is fast, easy, and doesn't require hospitalization or general sedation. This implies that the patient can continue typical exercises soon after the surgery. Furthermore, laser medical procedures are less intrusive than customary glaucoma medical procedures, which diminishes the risk of complexities like draining or contamination. Laser medical procedures likewise require less postoperative consideration and have a more limited recuperation time compared with other therapy choices.

The various kinds of laser medical procedures for glaucoma include Particular Laser Trabeculoplasty (SLT), Laser Fringe Iridotomy (LPI), and Transscleral Cyclophotocoagulation (TCP). Every one of these laser medical procedures has its own special approach to treating glaucoma and is resolved in light of the kind and severity of the glaucoma the patient has.

Particular Laser Trabeculoplasty (SLT) is a laser technique that focuses on the trabecular meshwork, the seepage arrangement of the eye. The laser utilized in the SLT strategy works by making minuscule changes to the meshwork to permit liquid to stream more effectively, decreasing eye pressure.

Laser Fringe Iridotomy (LPI) is one more kind of laser medical procedure for glaucoma that is utilized to treat point-conclusion glaucoma. The strategy works by making a little opening in the iris to permit liquid to stream all the more uninhibitedly. This kind of laser medical procedure can forestall future episodes of intense glaucoma assaults.

Transscleral Cyclophotocoagulation (TCP) is a more intrusive sort of laser medical procedure that is utilized to treat serious instances of glaucoma. The system includes utilizing a laser to obliterate a piece of the ciliary body, which produces watery humor (liquid in the eye). By obliterating a piece of the ciliary body, the technique lessens the development of watery humor, diminishing eye pressure in this manner.

Laser medical procedure for glaucoma is protected, yet likewise with any surgery, it conveys chances. Potential dangers include transitory increments for eye pressure, obscured vision, contamination, and dying. Patients who go through a laser medical procedure for glaucoma ought to adhere intently to their ophthalmologist's postoperative consideration directions and look for clinical consideration right away, assuming any side effects of contamination or confusion emerge.

13

Complementary therapies

Glaucoma is a difficult condition that influences the optic nerve and causes vision misfortune on the off chance that it is not treated quickly. This condition is generally brought about by the expanded tension in the eyes and is often connected with the development of liquid. Conventional clinical medicines normally incorporate the utilization of drugs and medical procedures, yet integral treatments can likewise be valuable for glaucoma patients. Integral treatments work to address basic needs, advance general wellbeing, and upgrade the impacts of regular medicines.

1. Acupuncture: Needle therapy is an old Chinese clinical practice that includes embedding needles into explicit places in the body. Needle therapy has been utilized to treat different ailments for millennia. In glaucoma, needle therapy assists with diminishing the strain in the eyes, further developing the bloodstream, and improving the progression of energy through the body. Needle therapy meetings ought to be done by an authorized acupuncturist.

2. Yoga: Yoga is a delicate type of activity that advances unwinding and decreases stress. This training additionally improves the blood stream and brings down the pulse, which can assist with lightening the side effects of glaucoma. Some yoga postures might in fact be performed while resting, which is ideal for glaucoma patients who need to abstain from twisting around or stressing.

3. Meditation: Contemplation is a superb method for quieting the psyche and diminishing pressure. Diminishing pressure is significant for individuals with glaucoma, as stress can increase strain in the eyes, demolishing the condition. Contemplation includes zeroing in on breathing or rehashing a word or expression to advance unwinding and work on general prosperity.

4. Diet and Nourishment: Appropriate nourishment is significant for overall well being, yet certain food sources can assist with easing

glaucoma side effects. Food sources that are wealthy in cell reinforcements and omega-3 unsaturated fats are advantageous for eye wellbeing and can assist with lessening strain in the eyes. An eating regimen that is rich in green, verdant vegetables, natural products, and nuts can likewise provide fundamental nutrients and supplements.

5. Rejuvenating balms: Medicinal oils can be utilized as an elective treatment for glaucoma. Rejuvenating oils like frankincense, cypress, and rosemary are accepted to decrease eye pressure and further develop vision. Natural balms can be utilized in a diffuser, weakened and applied topically, or ingested under the direction of an accomplished professional.

6. Homegrown Medication: Certain spices and enhancements have been displayed to assist with further developing eye wellbeing and decreasing glaucoma side effects. A few well-known natural solutions for glaucoma incorporate bilberry, ginkgo biloba, and curcumin. It is essential to talk with a certified medical care supplier prior to involving any natural cures or enhancements, as they might interface with different drugs or have side effects.

7. Mind-body treatment: Strategies like back rub treatment, Reiki, and reflexology can likewise assist glaucoma patients with lessening pressure and advancing unwinding. They can likewise further develop and lessen irritation in the eyes, which can ease glaucoma side effects.

IV

Living with Glaucoma

14

Coping strategies for those diagnosed

It is estimated that more than 3 million individuals in the US are affected by Glaucoma. The condition can be distressing and testing to make due, prompting a deficiency of personal satisfaction. Notwithstanding, there are viable survival techniques that people determined to have Glaucoma can use to live satisfying lives.

1. Get Educated

The most important phase in overseeing Glaucoma is to teach yourself about the illness. This can assist with diminishing nervousness, dread, and disarray surrounding the conclusion. You ought to comprehend how Glaucoma develops, its causes, risk variables, and treatment choices. There are a few assets accessible, for example, your ophthalmologist, support gatherings, or online discussions where you can accumulate data and interface with others going through exactly the same thing.

2. Establish a Good Relationship with Your Ophthalmologist

Having a good relationship with your ophthalmologist is fundamental while living with Glaucoma. Ordinary arrangements can assist you with dealing with the illness and identify any progressions sufficiently early to forestall further harm. It's fundamental to speak with your ophthalmologist about any worries or changes you might notice. They will likewise assist you with settling on the best treatment choices in light of your condition and phase of Glaucoma.

3. Adopt a Healthy Lifestyle

Keeping a sound way of life can help forestall and oversee Glaucoma. It incorporates a fair eating regimen, standard activity, getting satisfactory rest, abstaining from smoking, and lessening pressure. Practice increases the blood flow to the optic nerve and keeps up with, by and large, great wellbeing. Be that as it may, you ought to talk with your primary care physician prior to taking part in any actual work, as certain exercises may not be okay for people with Glaucoma.

4. Practice Good Eye Hygiene

Rehearsing great eye cleanliness is fundamental to overseeing Glaucoma. This includes cleaning your eyelids and lashes with warm water, abstaining from scouring your eyes, and utilizing defensive eyewear when essential. While cleaning up, utilize delicate, non-grating cleansers that don't disturb the eyes. Likewise, guarantee that your hands are spotless prior to touching your eyes to keep away from disease.

5. Use Visual Aids

Living with Glaucoma can sometimes bring about vision misfortune, which can influence your capacity to perform everyday exercises. Luckily, a few vision aids are accessible that can assist with working on your personal satisfaction. A few instances of vision help incorporate amplifying glasses, book recordings, talking watches, and PCs with huge screens. It's vital to talk with your ophthalmologist or optometrist to figure out which help will be best for you.

6. Join a Support Group.

Joining a care group for people with Glaucoma can be a superb method for tracking down solace, interacting with others going through comparable encounters, and offering data about survival techniques. You can learn from the encounters of others and gain an understanding of how to actually deal with the infection.

15

Rehabilitation services available

Luckily, there are restoration services accessible to assist those with glaucoma in dealing with their condition and keeping up with their vision. These services are presented by a range of experts, including ophthalmologists, optometrists, and word-related specialists. Some of the services that are accessible include:

1. Prescriptions: Glaucoma can be managed by utilizing medications, including eye drops. These drops work by diminishing the strain inside the eye, which is a significant risk factor for glaucoma. Now and again, patients might be prescribed pills to decrease their eye pressure.

2. Laser treatment: A few patients with glaucoma might be candidates for laser treatment. This includes utilizing a high-energy laser shaft to diminish the amount of liquid in the eye, which thus decreases pressure. Laser treatment should be possible in a short-term setting and regularly requires a couple of moments to finish.

3. Medical procedure: For certain patients, medical procedures might be important to oversee glaucoma. There are a few kinds of medical procedures that should be possible, including trabeculectomy, which includes making a little fold in the eye to deplete liquid, and shunting, which includes embedding a little gadget in the eye to assist with depleting liquid.

4. Occupational therapy: For those with glaucoma, it could be useful to work with a word-related advisor to learn better approaches for performing everyday assignments. Word-related treatment can assist patients with keeping up with their autonomy and working on their personal satisfaction.

5. Low vision services: For people who have encountered critical vision misfortune because of glaucoma, low vision services might be useful. These administrations can incorporate assistive gadgets like magnifiers as well as teach how to utilize them.

Rehabilitation services can be a pivotal piece of overseeing glaucoma. These administrations can assist patients with keeping up with their vision, dealing with their condition, and working on their personal satisfaction. Assuming you or somebody you love has been diagnosed to have glaucoma, it is essential to converse with your primary care physician about what restoration administrations might be accessible and suitable for your requirements. By cooperating, you can assist with dealing with this condition and keep up with your vision as far as might be feasible.

16

Lifestyle changes to manage Glaucoma

An extensive treatment plan for glaucoma can incorporate lifestyle changes.

One way of life change that can assist with overseeing glaucoma is by maintaining a sound eating routine. As indicated by research, supplements like nutrients A, C, and E are fundamental for the legitimate working of the eyes. Moreover, expanding the intake of leafy foods can further develop eye wellbeing, which can postpone the development of glaucoma. Eating foods high in sound fats, for example, Omega-3 unsaturated fats, can assist with forestalling further vision misfortune. Subsequently, making changes to your eating regimen to incorporate more vegetables, organic products, and solid fats can have an effect.

Another way of life change that can assist with overseeing glaucoma is by practicing consistently. Research demonstrates that exercise assists in increasing the blood flow in the body, which incorporates the eyes, diminishing intraocular pressure, which is a risk factor for glaucoma. Oxygen-consuming activities like strolling, swimming, cycling, and running for somewhere around thirty minutes every day can fundamentally assist with overseeing glaucoma. It is fundamental to keep away from high-influence sports, like boxing and hard work, as these exercises can make the eye go through pressure changes, which can increment intraocular pressure, prompting optic nerve harm.

Stressed executives can likewise assist with overseeing glaucoma. Studies recommend that feelings of anxiety and the intraocular strain in the eye are connected. Subsequently, embracing methods that can lessen feelings of anxiety, like yoga, contemplation, or profound breathing, can be viable in overseeing glaucoma. One can join yoga or contemplation classes or partake in exercises, for example, kendo or fragrance-based treatments, to actually manage feelings of anxiety.

Overseeing eye care and medicine routines is another pivotal way of life change in overseeing glaucoma. Individuals who have glaucoma need to go through routine eye assessments at regular intervals to screen for the condition and guarantee it is taken care of. It is likewise urgent to stick to the recommended drug regimen and to guarantee that one accepts the right measurements as endorsed. Conflicting prescription routines and ill-advised utilization of eye drops can deteriorate glaucoma, prompting vision misfortune. Setting a suggestion to take the medicine, following the right measurements, and following the drug's directions are important to forestall further inconveniences.

Moreover, one can safeguard their eyes by making small but significant lifestyle changes, for example, wearing shades that shield the eyes from the sun's destructive beams, wearing goggles during exercises, for example, swimming or home improvement exercises that can open the eyes to synthetics or particles, and getting sufficient rest to rest the eyes.

Lifestyle changes like solid eating routine decisions, standard workout schedules, reducing stress across the board, and routine eye care and medicine regimens can assist with overseeing glaucoma. Little changes like wearing shades and goggles or getting sufficient rest can likewise shield the eyes from harm.

17

Conclusion

Glaucoma, the subsequent driving reason for visual deficiency around the world, is a quiet cheat that can deny us our vision without giving any early advance notice indications. Unlike other eye conditions, like cataracts and macular degeneration, glaucoma commonly has no apparent side effects until it has advanced to a high-level stage, making early identification and avoidance fundamental.

While the specific reason for glaucoma remains obscure, specialists concur that the risk factors incorporate age, family ancestry, hypertension, diabetes, and certain prescriptions. Hence, assuming you have any of these risk factors, you ought to ensure that you get your customary eye tests.

Fortunately, you can forestall glaucoma and safeguard your visual perception by making some lifestyle changes and taking on sound propensities.

1. Get Standard Eye Tests: The most important stage in preventing glaucoma is getting standard eye tests. Specialists suggest having your eyes checked every one to two years, particularly on the off chance that you have a family history of glaucoma or any of the risk factors referenced previously. An eye test can recognize early indications of glaucoma before it becomes irreversible.

2. Deal with Your Wellbeing: Glaucoma is related to a few fundamental ailments, for example, hypertension and diabetes. In this way, dealing with these circumstances is vital to forestalling glaucoma. Keep your circulatory strain and glucose levels under control by eating a sound diet, practicing routinely, and accepting your prescriptions as endorsed.

3. Safeguard Your Eyes from UV Beams: Openness to bright (UV) radiation can increase your risk of fostering specific eye conditions, including glaucoma. In this manner, it is fundamental to shield your eyes from UV beams by wearing shades with 100 percent UV security at whatever point you are outside during the day.

4. Stop Smoking: Smoking is a huge risk factor for glaucoma, as it can harm the optic nerve and increase eye pressure. On the off chance that you smoke, quit as quickly as time permits, and in the event that you don't smoke, don't begin.

5. Limit Caffeine and Liquor: Polishing off an excess of caffeine and liquor can build your eye pressure, making you more vulnerable to glaucoma. Thusly, it is ideal to restrict your admission of these substances and select better drinks, all things being equal.

6. Work out regularly: Ordinary activity helps your general wellbeing as well as forestall glaucoma. Exercise can assist with bringing down your intraocular pressure (IOP), a main risk factor for glaucoma, by expanding the bloodstream and diminishing irritation.

7. Follow a Solid Eating routine: Eating a sound eating regimen rich in organic products, vegetables, and omega-3 unsaturated fats can assist with forestalling glaucoma. These supplements have cell reinforcement and calming properties that shield the eyes from harm brought about by oxidative pressure.

Glaucoma prevention ought to be a first concern for everybody, particularly those with risk factors. Early discovery and treatment are pivotal in forestalling the movement of glaucoma and saving your visual perception.

In any case, there are a few counteraction systems and sound propensities that people can take on to decrease the risk of creating glaucoma.

1. Regular Eye Tests

One of the main prevention procedures for glaucoma is to have standard eye tests. People beyond 40 years old have a thorough eye test every 1-2 years. This takes into consideration the early location of any potential eye illnesses, including glaucoma, and guarantees convenient therapy to forestall long-lasting harm to the optic nerve.

2. Manage chronic conditions

Overseeing ongoing circumstances, for example, diabetes and hypertension, can likewise decrease the risk of creating glaucoma. People with these circumstances ought to heed their primary care physician's guidance in regards to eating less, exercising, and medicine to keep up with their overall wellbeing and forestall further difficulties.

3. Keep a Sound Eating regimen.

A sound eating regimen can likewise play a part in forestalling glaucoma. Research has shown that food varieties rich in cell reinforcements, like products of the soil, can shield the optic nerve from harm. Specifically, salad greens like kale, spinach, and collard greens are particularly helpful because of their high levels of lutein and zeaxanthin, two cell reinforcements that are significant for eye wellbeing.

4. Work out consistently.

Practice is fundamental for overall wellbeing and can likewise be useful for eye wellbeing. Moderate actual work like strolling, cycling, or swimming for no less than 30 minutes daily can diminish intraocular pressure, a key risk factor for glaucoma.

5. Try not to smoke.

Smoking is a huge risk factor for different infections, including glaucoma. Smokers are twice as likely to foster glaucoma as non-smokers. Stopping smoking can lessen this gamble and, furthermore, give numerous other medical advantages.

6. Wear protective eyewear.

Defensive eyewear, for example, goggles or security glasses, can forestall eye wounds that can prompt glaucoma. These wounds can happen during sports, yard work, or different exercises where items might come into contact with the eye.

7. Manage Pressure

Stress can likewise adversely affect eye wellbeing and increase the risk of developing glaucoma. Participating in unwinding strategies like contemplation, yoga, or profound breathing activities can decrease feelings of anxiety and, generally speaking, advance prosperity.

Preventing glaucoma requires embracing a mix of solid propensities and counteraction systems. Normal eye tests, overseeing ongoing circumstances, keeping a sound eating routine, practicing consistently, abstaining from smoking, wearing defensive eyewear, and overseeing pressure are all fundamental advances that people can require to diminish their risk of fostering this serious eye sickness. By integrating these propensities into their day-to-day daily practice, people can safeguard their vision and appreciate ideal eye wellbeing all through their lifetime.

Dealing with our eyes is quite possibly one of the most vital steps we can take towards our general prosperity. Our eyes permit us to see our general surroundings, assisting us in exploring our environmental elements and experiencing life's little delights. However, in spite of its importance, a great many people will generally neglect their eye health. We frequently focus on different parts of our prosperity, like our actual wellness or diet, while overlooking our eye care needs. This disregard could prompt a few issues that can influence our day-to-day routines, like unfortunate vision or eye diseases.

The following are a couple of things we can do to assume responsibility for our eye's wellbeing:

1. Get standard eye tests.

Standard eye tests are quite possibly the main thing we can do to keep up with solid eyes. Your optometrist or ophthalmologist can recognize early indications of eye issues like glaucoma, waterfalls, and age-related macular degeneration before they progress into additional difficult issues. You ought to plan customary eye tests every one to two years, contingent upon your age, family ancestry, and clinical history.

2. Maintain a healthy lifestyle.

A few investigations have shown that lifestyle factors like activity, diet, and rest can influence our visual perception. By eating a sound and adjusted diet and remembering food sources rich in nutrients A, C, and E and omega-3 unsaturated fats, we can further develop our eye wellbeing. Additionally, engaging in ordinary active work and getting sufficient rest can further develop blood flow and lessen the risk of creating eye-related issues.

3. Wear protective eyewear.

Our eyes are defenseless to different ecological factors like residue, sun, and synthetics. Wearing defensive eyewear, for example, shades, security glasses, or goggles, can forestall wounds and long-term harm to our eyes. These eyewear items are effectively available and reasonable, so there is no justification for not wearing them.

4. Practice good eye hygiene.

Pursuing great eye hygiene routines can forestall the spread of eye diseases. Cleaning up prior to contacting our eyes and not sharing towels or cosmetics can fundamentally decrease the risk of contamination. Additionally, abstaining from scouring our eyes, eliminating our contact focal points before bed, and not utilizing terminated eye drops or arrangements can prevent different eye-related issues.

5. Educate others

By teaching others about the significance of dealing with our eyes, we can have a huge effect. Spreading mindfulness about the advantages of ordinary eye tests and solid way of life propensities can urge individuals to focus on their eye wellbeing. We can do this by sharing articles and online journals like this one, making virtual entertainment posts, and beginning discussions with our loved ones.

Dealing with our eye health ought to be a fundamental piece of our daily schedule.

Made in United States
Troutdale, OR
03/16/2024

18521071R00030